The Ayurvedic Guide to Healthy Hair

"Treating Hair Loss Naturally"

Peter Miller

Table Of Content

INTRODUCTION

The Ayurvedic Guide to Healthy Hair: Treating Hair Loss Naturally is a comprehensive guide to using Ayurvedic principles and remedies to address hair loss and promote healthy hair growth. Ayurveda is an ancient system of medicine that originated in India and is based on the belief that health and wellness depend on a delicate balance between the mind, body, and spirit.

Hair loss is a common concern that affects many people, regardless of age, gender, or ethnicity. The reasons for hair loss are many, including genetics, hormonal changes, stress, poor diet, and certain medical conditions. While conventional treatments for hair loss often involve the use of drugs and surgery, these methods can be costly and come with potential side effects.

The Ayurvedic approach to hair loss is different. It recognizes that hair loss is often a symptom of an underlying imbalance in the body and seeks to address the root cause of the problem. Ayurveda uses a holistic approach to health that includes dietary changes, herbal remedies, and lifestyle modifications to restore balance and promote optimal health.

This book provides a detailed overview of the Ayurvedic approach to hair loss, including the causes of hair loss and the Ayurvedic principles that underlie treatment. The book also includes a variety of Ayurvedic remedies for hair loss, including dietary changes, herbal supplements, and topical treatments. Whether you're just starting to experience hair loss or have been struggling with it for some time, this book offers practical and effective solutions to help you achieve healthy, vibrant hair.

CHAPTER ONE
Understanding Hair Loss in Ayurveda

Hair loss is a common concern that affects many people, regardless of age, gender, or ethnicity. While conventional treatments for hair loss often involve the use of drugs and surgery, these methods can be costly and come with potential side effects. The Ayurvedic approach to hair loss is different, recognizing that hair loss is often a symptom of an underlying imbalance in the body and seeking to address the root cause of the problem. In this chapter, we will explore the basics of Ayurveda and hair loss and the Ayurvedic perspective on the causes of hair loss.

Introduction to Ayurveda:

Ayurveda is an ancient system of medicine that originated in India and is based on the belief that health and wellness depend on a delicate balance between the mind, body, and spirit. The Ayurvedic approach to health is holistic and seeks to address not just physical symptoms, but also the underlying emotional and spiritual factors that contribute to imbalance. Ayurveda uses a variety of tools and techniques to restore balance, including dietary changes, herbal remedies, and lifestyle modifications.

Causes of hair loss and the Ayurvedic perspective:

In Ayurveda, hair loss is often seen as a symptom of an underlying imbalance in the body, such as an imbalance in the three doshas, or the energies that govern our physical, mental, and emotional well-being. Some of the most common causes of hair loss in Ayurveda include stress, poor diet, hormonal changes, and certain medical conditions. In order to effectively address hair loss, Ayurveda seeks to identify and address the root cause of the imbalance, rather than simply treating the symptom.

Understanding the three doshas and their impact on hair health:

The three doshas in Ayurveda are vata, pitta, and kapha, and each has a unique impact on hair health. Vata governs movement and circulation in the body, including blood flow to the scalp, and an imbalance in vata can lead to dry, brittle hair and hair loss. Pitta governs metabolism and digestion, and an imbalance in pitta can lead to inflammation and hair loss. Kapha governs structure and stability in the body, and an imbalance in kapha can lead to heavy, greasy hair and hair loss. By understanding the impact of each dosha on hair health, it is possible to develop an Ayurvedic treatment plan that addresses the root cause of the imbalance.

In conclusion, this chapter serves as an introduction to the Ayurvedic approach to hair loss, including the causes of hair loss and the Ayurvedic perspective on the root causes of imbalance. By understanding the impact of the three doshas on hair health, it is possible to develop a personalized treatment plan that addresses the root cause of hair loss and promotes healthy hair growth.

CHAPTER TWO
The Ayurvedic Diet for Healthy Hair

A balanced diet is essential for good health and wellness in Ayurveda, and this is particularly true for the health of your hair. The food you eat provides the nutrients that your hair needs to grow and stay strong, and an imbalanced diet can lead to hair loss and other hair problems. In this chapter, we will explore the importance of a balanced diet in Ayurveda and the foods you should include and avoid for healthy hair.

Importance of a balanced diet in Ayurveda:

In Ayurveda, a balanced diet is seen as one of the most important factors in maintaining good health and wellness. A balanced diet should provide all the nutrients the body needs to function properly, including vitamins, minerals, and essential fatty acids. By eating a balanced diet, you can help to restore balance to the body and prevent imbalances that can lead to hair loss and other hair problems.

Foods to include and avoid for healthy hair:

In Ayurveda, there are certain foods that are recommended for healthy hair and others that are best avoided. Foods to include in your diet for healthy hair include dark leafy greens, nuts and seeds, fatty fish, and eggs. These foods are rich in vitamins, minerals, and essential fatty acids that are essential for healthy hair growth. Foods to avoid for healthy hair include processed foods, sugar, and refined carbohydrates, as these can lead to inflammation and an imbalance in the body.

Ayurvedic dietary recommendations for hair loss:

In addition to eating a balanced diet that includes the right foods for healthy hair, there are specific Ayurvedic dietary recommendations for hair loss. For example, it is recommended to eat warm, cooked foods that are easy to digest, as this can help to reduce stress on the body and promote healthy hair growth. Herbs such as fenugreek, amla, and Brahmi are also recommended for their ability to support healthy hair growth.

This chapter highlights the importance of a balanced diet in Ayurveda and the role of food in maintaining healthy hair. By including the right foods in your diet and avoiding those that can lead to imbalances, you can help to promote healthy hair growth and prevent hair loss. By following the Ayurvedic dietary recommendations for hair loss, you can support your body in its natural ability to heal and maintain healthy hair.

CHAPTER THREE
Herbs and Supplements for Hair Loss

Ayurveda has a rich tradition of using herbs and supplements to promote hair health and treat hair loss. In this chapter, we will explore the various Ayurvedic herbs and supplements that are used to promote hair growth and reduce hair loss. We will also discuss dosage, administration, and safety considerations for these remedies.

Overview of Ayurvedic herbs for hair health:

Ayurveda has a long tradition of using herbs to promote hair health and treat hair loss. Some of the most commonly used Ayurvedic herbs for hair health include amla, Brahmi, fenugreek, licorice root, and hibiscus. These herbs are believed to promote hair growth, reduce hair loss, and improve the overall health of the scalp and hair.

Herbs for promoting hair growth and reducing hair loss:

Amla, Brahmi, and fenugreek are some of the most commonly used Ayurvedic herbs for promoting hair growth and reducing hair loss. Amla is rich in antioxidants and is believed to support healthy hair growth by strengthening the hair shaft. Brahmi is thought to improve blood circulation to the scalp and promote hair growth, while fenugreek is believed to provide essential nutrients to the hair and scalp, helping to prevent hair loss.

Dosage, administration, and safety considerations for Ayurvedic herbs:

When using Ayurvedic herbs for hair loss, it is important to follow the recommended dosages and administration methods. Some herbs, such as amla and fenugreek, can be consumed in supplement form or applied topically to the hair and scalp. Others, such as Brahmi, may be taken in capsule or tincture form. Before using any Ayurvedic herbs, it is important to consult with a qualified Ayurvedic practitioner to ensure the correct dosage and administration methods for your specific needs. Additionally, it is important to consider any potential side effects or interactions with other medications, as some Ayurvedic herbs may not be safe for everyone.

This chapter highlights the various Ayurvedic herbs and supplements that can be used to promote hair health and treat hair loss. By understanding the different herbs and their benefits, as well as their dosage, administration, and safety considerations, you can make informed choices about which remedies may be right for you. With the right combination of diet, herbs, and supplements, you can support your body in its natural ability to maintain healthy hair and reduce hair loss.

CHAPTER FOUR
Topical Treatments for Hair Loss

In addition to dietary changes and herbal supplements, topical treatments can also play an important role in promoting hair health and treating hair loss in Ayurveda. In this chapter, we will explore the different Ayurvedic oils and hair masks that can be used to support healthy hair and reduce hair loss.

Ayurvedic oils for healthy hair:
Ayurvedic oils are a staple in the treatment of hair loss in Ayurveda. Some of the most commonly used oils include coconut oil, castor oil, and sesame oil. These oils are believed to moisturize the scalp and hair, promote blood circulation to the scalp, and nourish the hair shaft, helping to prevent hair loss and promote healthy hair growth.

Homemade Ayurvedic hair masks and treatments:
In addition to oils, there are a number of Ayurvedic hair masks and treatments that

can be made at home to support healthy hair. Some popular ingredients in Ayurvedic hair masks include aloe vera, henna, and fenugreek. These ingredients are believed to promote hair growth, reduce hair loss, and improve the overall health of the scalp and hair.

The benefits and use of Ayurvedic hair oils:

Ayurvedic hair oils are believed to offer a number of benefits for healthy hair. For example, coconut oil is believed to moisturize the hair and scalp, preventing dryness, and promoting healthy hair growth. Castor oil is believed to promote blood circulation to the scalp and nourish the hair shaft, helping to prevent hair loss. To use Ayurvedic hair oils, they can be applied to the scalp and hair, left in for a specified period of time, and then washed out with a mild shampoo.

In conclusion, topical treatments such as Ayurvedic oils and hair masks can be an effective way to support healthy hair and reduce hair loss in Ayurveda. By incorporating these remedies into your hair care routine, you can help to nourish your scalp and hair, promoting healthy hair growth and reducing hair loss.

CHAPTER FIVE
Lifestyle Changes for Healthy Hair

In this chapter, we will explore the impact of stress and other lifestyle factors on hair health and how incorporating Ayurvedic practices and changes can help promote healthy hair growth and reduce hair loss.

The impact of stress on hair health:
Stress is a known trigger for hair loss and can have a significant impact on hair health. In Ayurveda, stress is believed to increase the production of cortisol, a hormone that can cause hair loss and damage to the hair follicles. Furthermore, stress can also disrupt the balance of the doshas, leading to further hair loss and damage.

Ayurvedic practices for reducing stress and promoting hair health:
There are a number of Ayurvedic practices that can be used to reduce stress and promote hair health. Some of these practices include meditation, yoga, and pranayama

(breathing exercises). These practices are believed to calm the mind, reduce stress levels, and promote overall hair health.

Exercise, sleep, and other lifestyle changes for optimal hair health:

In addition to Ayurvedic practices, there are a number of other lifestyle changes that can help promote optimal hair health. Regular exercise and getting adequate sleep are two important factors that can impact hair health. Exercise can promote blood flow to the scalp, while adequate sleep can help reduce stress levels and promote overall health. Other lifestyle changes that can impact hair health include reducing alcohol and caffeine intake, avoiding harsh hair treatments, and managing any medical conditions that may be contributing to hair loss.

Conclusion: In this chapter, we have explored the impact of stress and other lifestyle factors on hair health and how incorporating Ayurvedic practices and changes can help promote healthy hair growth and reduce hair loss. Making small changes to your lifestyle, incorporating Ayurvedic practices, and reducing stress levels can all contribute to a healthier head of hair. As always, it's important to consult with a healthcare professional before making any changes to your routine, especially if you have any medical conditions or are taking any medications.

CHAPTER SIX
Combining Ayurvedic Principles for Optimal Hair Health

In this chapter, we will explore how to integrate Ayurvedic principles for the best results when treating hair loss. We will also discuss how to personalize your Ayurvedic approach to achieve optimal hair health and how to maintain hair health with regular Ayurvedic practices.

Integrating Ayurvedic principles for the best results:

In order to achieve optimal hair health, it is important to integrate a variety of Ayurvedic principles. This includes incorporating the right diet, herbal supplements, topical treatments, and lifestyle changes into your routine. Each of these factors can contribute to the overall health of your hair, and by combining them, you can maximize their benefits.

Personalizing your Ayurvedic approach to hair loss:

Every individual is unique, and so is their hair loss. It's important to understand your own unique constitution and the underlying cause of your hair loss in order to determine the best approach for treating it. A qualified Ayurvedic practitioner can help you identify the root cause of your hair loss and develop a personalized plan to help restore your hair health.

Maintaining hair health with regular Ayurvedic practices:

Maintaining healthy hair requires a long-term commitment to incorporating Ayurvedic principles into your routine. This includes regular use of Ayurvedic oils, herbal supplements, and topical treatments, as well as making healthy lifestyle choices, such as reducing stress, getting adequate sleep, and eating a balanced diet. By regularly incorporating these Ayurvedic practices into your routine, you can help maintain optimal hair health for the long term.

We have explored how to integrate Ayurvedic principles for the best results when treating hair loss, how to personalize your Ayurvedic approach to achieve optimal hair health, and how to maintain hair health with regular Ayurvedic practices. By following these principles and incorporating Ayurvedic practices into your routine, you can help achieve and maintain optimal hair health for the long term.

CHAPTER SEVEN
Managing Hair Loss in Women

Hair loss is a common concern for both men and women, but the causes and treatment options can differ between the sexes. In this chapter, we will focus on the specific challenges faced by women when it comes to hair loss and how Ayurveda can be used to manage this condition.

Understanding the causes of hair loss in women:

Hair loss in women can be caused by a variety of factors, including hormonal changes, stress, dietary deficiencies, and certain medical conditions. In some cases, hair loss can also be a side effect of certain medications. Understanding the underlying cause of your hair loss is key to developing an effective treatment plan.

Ayurvedic treatments for hair loss in women:

Ayurveda offers a number of effective treatments for hair loss in women, including dietary changes, herbal supplements, topical treatments, and lifestyle changes. By addressing the root cause of your hair loss, Ayurveda can help to promote hair growth and restore hair health.

Managing hormonal changes:

Hormonal changes, such as those that occur during menopause, can have a significant impact on hair health. Ayurveda offers a number of natural remedies to help manage these changes and promote healthy hair growth, including dietary changes, herbal supplements, and topical treatments.

Stress management:

Stress is a common cause of hair loss in women and can have a significant impact on hair health. Ayurveda offers a number of stress-management techniques, including meditation, yoga, and aromatherapy, to help reduce stress and promote hair health.

Hair loss is a common concern for women, but Ayurveda offers a number of effective treatments to help manage this condition. By addressing the root cause of your hair loss, incorporating Ayurvedic dietary changes, herbal supplements, topical treatments, and lifestyle changes into your routine, you can help to promote hair growth and restore hair health. By following these principles, you can help to achieve and maintain optimal hair health for the long term.

CHAPTER EIGHT
Managing Hair Loss in Men

Hair loss is a common concern for both men and women, but the causes and treatment options can differ between the sexes. In this chapter, we will focus on the specific challenges faced by men when it comes to hair loss and how Ayurveda can be used to manage this condition.

Understanding the causes of male-pattern hair loss:

Male-pattern hair loss is the most common cause of hair loss in men and is caused by a combination of genetics and hormones. Understanding the underlying cause of your hair loss is key to developing an effective treatment plan.

Ayurvedic remedies for male-pattern hair loss:

Ayurveda offers a number of effective remedies for male-pattern hair loss, including dietary changes, herbal supplements, topical treatments, and lifestyle changes. By addressing the root cause of your hair loss, Ayurveda can help to promote hair growth and restore hair health.

Herbs and supplements for healthy hair:

Ayurveda offers a number of herbs and supplements that are known to promote hair growth and reduce hair loss. Some of the most commonly used herbs for hair health include ashwagandha, bhringraj, and amla.

Lifestyle changes for optimal hair health:

In addition to dietary changes and herbal remedies, Ayurveda also emphasizes the importance of making lifestyle changes for optimal hair health. This may include reducing stress, getting adequate sleep, and engaging in regular physical activity.

Hair loss is a common concern for men, but Ayurveda offers a number of effective treatments to help manage this condition. By addressing the root cause of your hair loss and incorporating Ayurvedic dietary changes, herbal supplements, topical treatments, and lifestyle changes into your routine, you can help to promote hair growth and restore hair health. By following these principles, you can help to achieve and maintain optimal hair health for the long term.

CHAPTER NINE
Tips for Maintaining Healthy Hair

In this chapter, we will focus on the tips and habits that can help you maintain healthy hair and prevent hair loss. Maintaining the health of your hair requires not just the right diet and topical treatments, but also making some changes to your daily habits.

Daily Habits for Healthy Hair:

Maintaining a healthy and balanced diet is crucial for healthy hair, but there are other things you can do every day to keep your hair in top condition. These include:

- Avoiding harsh chemicals and heat styling: Harsh chemicals like hair dyes, bleach, and straightening agents can damage your hair, making it dry and brittle. Similarly, excessive heat styling, such as flat ironing or blow-drying, can also harm your hair. Consider using natural and mild products and limit the use of heat styling.

- Brushing your hair gently: Brushing your hair too vigorously or using a brush with stiff bristles can cause breakage and tangles. Use a wide-toothed comb or brush to detangle your hair gently, starting from the ends and working your way up to the roots.

- Protecting your hair from the sun and wind: Just like your skin, your hair can also be damaged by excessive sun exposure and wind. Consider wearing a hat or scarf to protect your hair when you're out in the sun and avoid sleeping with your hair loose if it tends to get tangled at night.

Avoiding Common Hair Care Mistakes: In addition to the habits mentioned above, there are some common mistakes that you should avoid to keep your hair healthy. These include:

- Overwashing: Overwashing your hair can strip it of its natural oils, leaving it dry and brittle. Wash your hair only when it's necessary, and use a mild, nourishing shampoo and conditioner.

- Skipping regular trims: Regular trims are important for maintaining the health of your hair, as they remove split ends and damaged hair.

Maintaining Hair Health with Regular Ayurvedic Practices:

In addition to the tips mentioned above, incorporating regular Ayurvedic practices into your routine can help you maintain healthy hair and prevent hair loss. These include:

- Using Ayurvedic oils and herbs: Regular use of Ayurvedic oils and herbs can promote healthy hair growth and prevent hair loss.

- Following a balanced Ayurvedic diet: Eating a balanced diet that includes all the nutrients your hair needs can help keep it healthy and strong.

- Incorporating stress-reducing practices: Stress can have a negative impact on your hair health, so it's important to find ways to reduce stress in your life. Incorporating stress-reducing practices like meditation, yoga, or deep breathing into your routine can help you keep your hair healthy and strong.

CHAPTER TEN
Conclusion and Final Thoughts

In this chapter, we will bring together the key points covered in the book and provide some final thoughts and encouragement for your journey to healthy hair through Ayurveda.

Recap of Key Points:

In this section, we will summarize the main principles and practices discussed in the book, highlighting the most important aspects of Ayurvedic hair loss treatment. This will help reinforce the information you have learned and provide a convenient reference guide for future use.

Maintaining Hair Health for the Long Term:

We will also discuss the importance of maintaining hair health for the long term, offering practical tips and suggestions for incorporating Ayurvedic principles into your daily routine. This will help you achieve and maintain healthy, strong, and radiant hair for years to come.

Encouragement and Support for Your Ayurvedic Journey:

Finally, we will offer encouragement and support for your Ayurvedic journey to healthy hair. We understand that making changes to your hair care routine and lifestyle can be challenging, but with the right guidance and support, it is possible to achieve the healthy, beautiful hair you desire. We will provide inspiration and guidance to help you stay motivated and on track.

This book has provided a comprehensive guide to Ayurvedic hair loss treatment, covering the key principles, practices, and habits that can help you achieve healthy, strong, and radiant hair. We hope that this book has provided valuable insights and practical tips to help you on your journey to healthy hair through Ayurveda.